ouijdane bk

JANA AT THE HOSPITAL

DIARY OF JANA

It is 8 pm, but Jana can't sleep tonight. she can feel the pain in her throat again. She thought the pain will never come back.

The doctor comes to examine Jana who is laying down on her bed, closing her eyes, and waiting for the pain to go away.

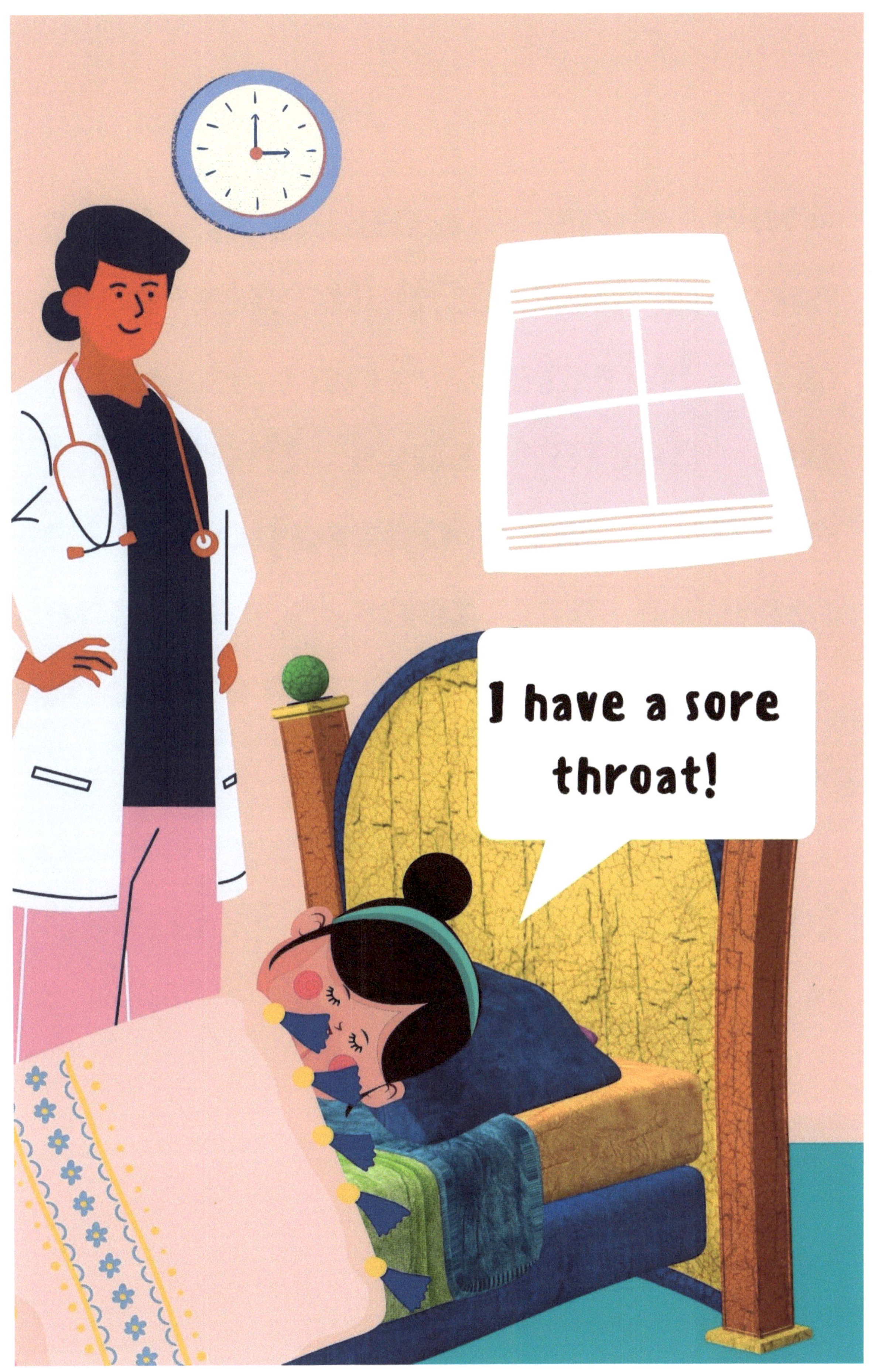
I have a sore throat!

Jana has **tonsillitis**; this means her tonsils get sore and infected. That is why the doctor says that she needs an operation to remove her tonsils, so she will not have sorethroat again.

The surgery to remove tonsils is called a **tonsillectomy**.

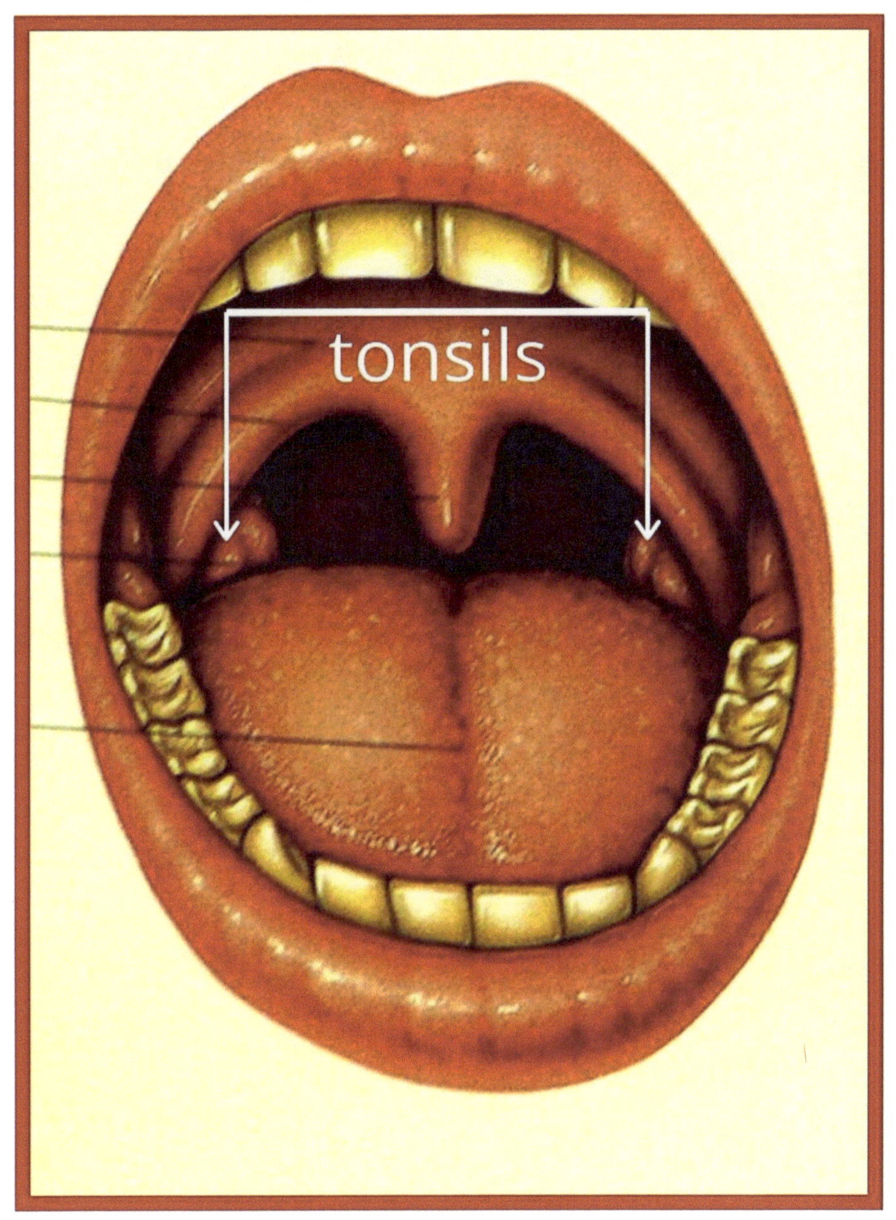

tonsils

Jana is scared, and as she has never been to the hospital for a surgery, she has a lot of questions:

how do doctors get the tonsils out of her throat? Will it hurt?
And what exactly do tonsils do back there?

The doctor promises to answer all the questions, but first of all Jana needs to understand the reason why she will do this surgery, in order to overcome her fear. Her parents and the doctor want to help her get better, and Jana wants to stop the pain so she can go to the school, play with her friends, and eat the meals she loves.

The night before surgery, Jana is not allowed to eat or drink anything after dinner, because her stomach must be empty for surgery.

Today is the day of the surgery, Jana and her mom are packing the suitcase, she can bring anything she wants to have with her; her prefered book and her lovely teddy bear. It's nice to have something that reminds you of home when you're in the hospital.

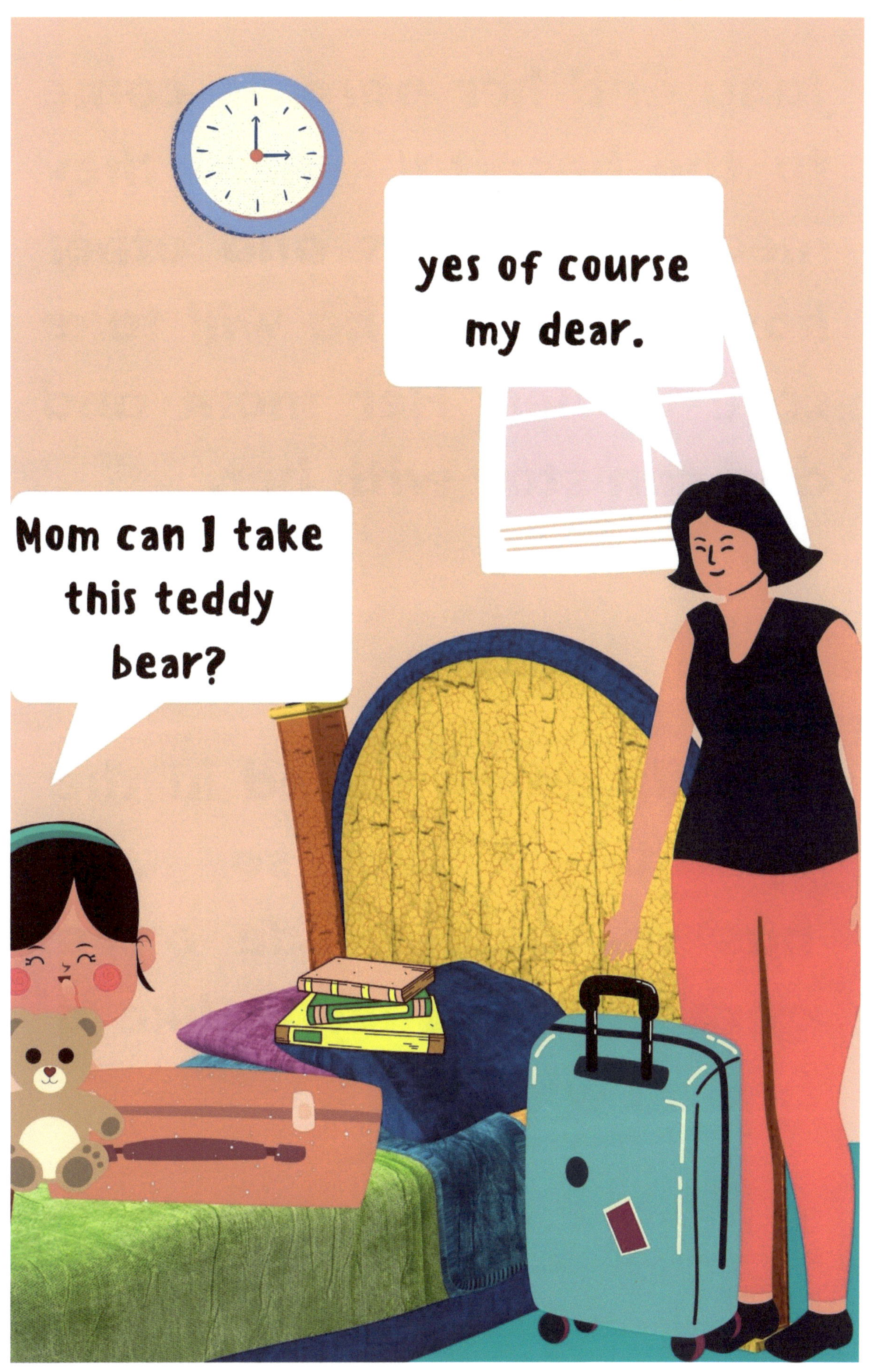
yes of course my dear.
Mom can I take this teddy bear?

Jana and her parents come to the hospital where they meet the nurses and other hospital staff who will take care of her. Her mom and dad can stay with her.

Tonsils are removed in the operating room, so Jana has to take a ride on a gurney. A gurney is like a bed on wheels.

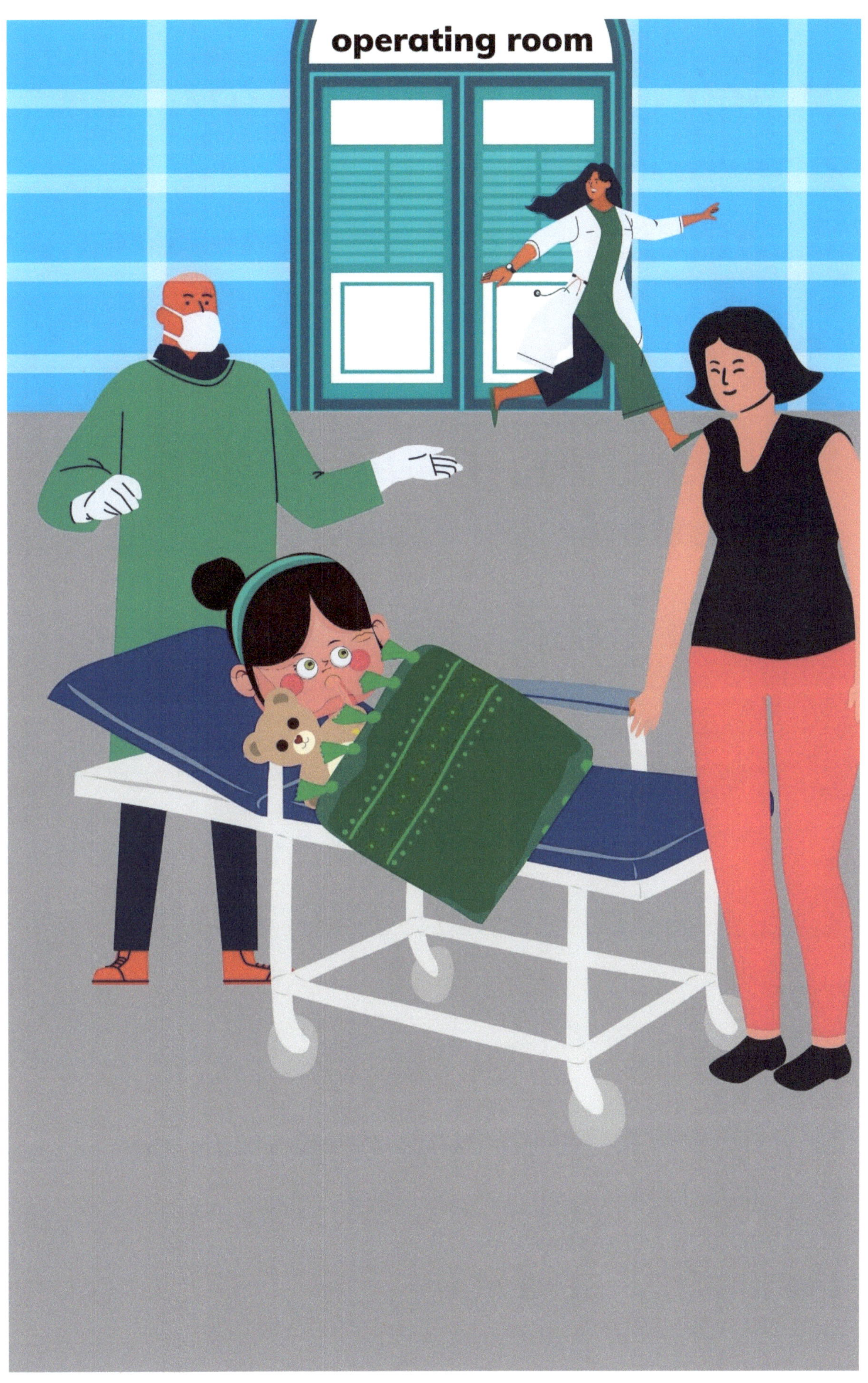
operating room

When it's time for her operation, Jana gets
a medicine called anesthesia that will help her fall asleep and keep her from
feeling any pain during the operation.

During the surgery, which takes only about 20 minutes, doctors open Jana's mouth and remove the tonsils. Jana does not feel anything during the
operation because she is sleeping. Before she know it, she will wake up in the recovery room.

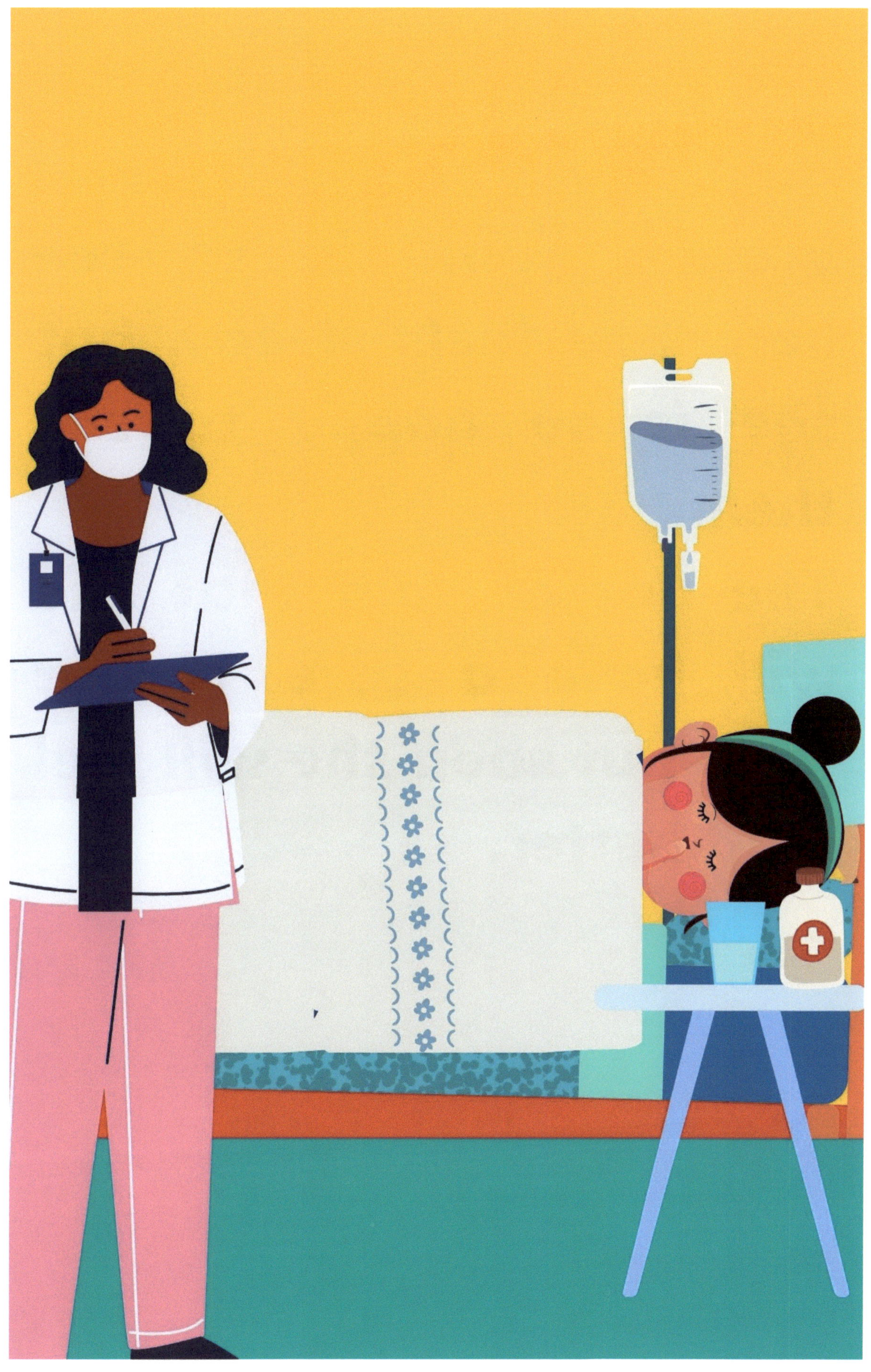

Jana's mom, dad, and brother come in to see her. She feels sleepy, but she is so happy to see them.
The doctor said that she will have a sore Throat first. But soon she will feel a lot better.

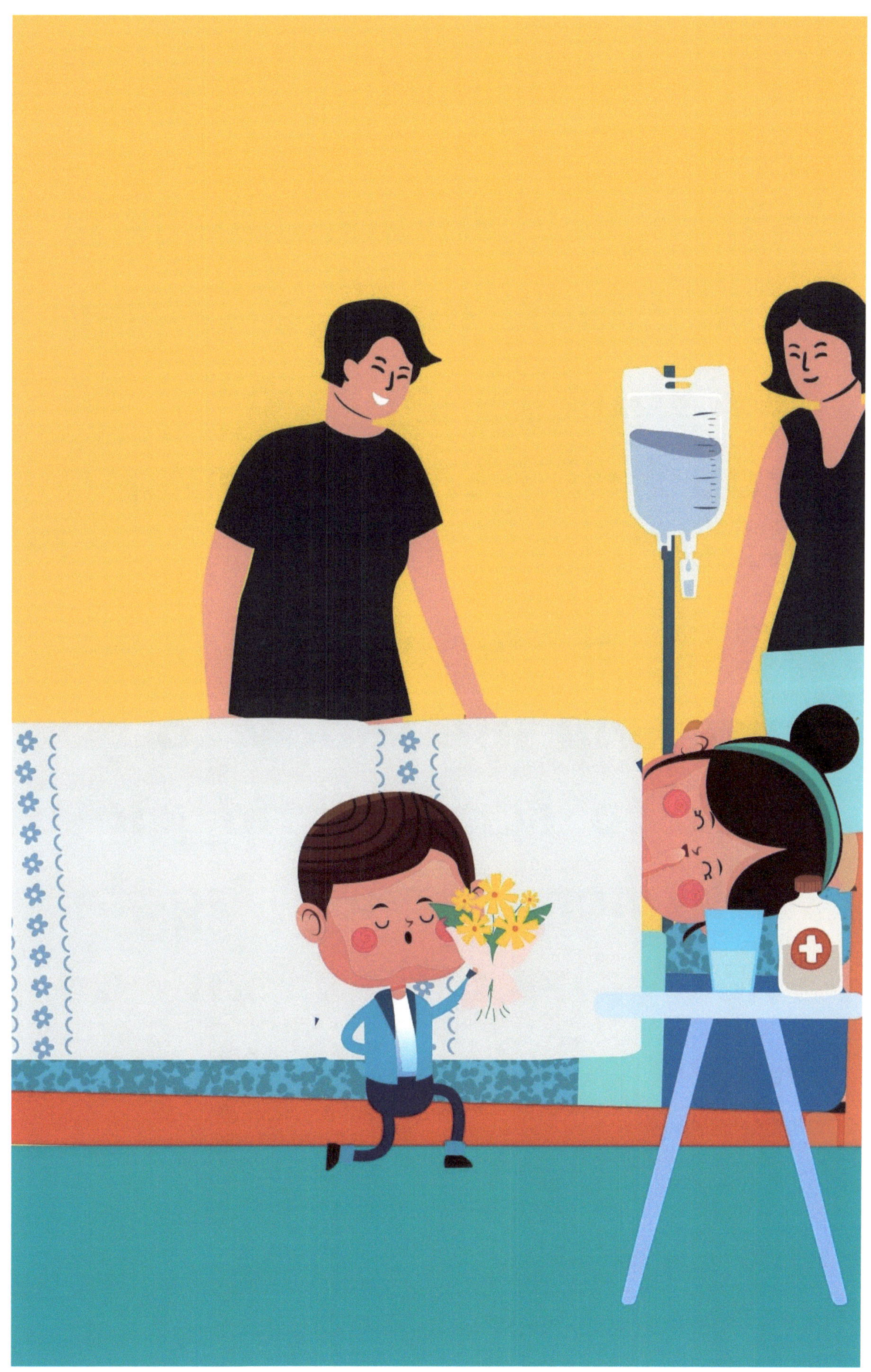

When her doctor say it is okay, Jana can go home. Everyone will be so proud of her for doing a great job!

After a week or two, Jana will be ready to go back to school and play with her friends again. She can tell them all about her tonsillectomy!

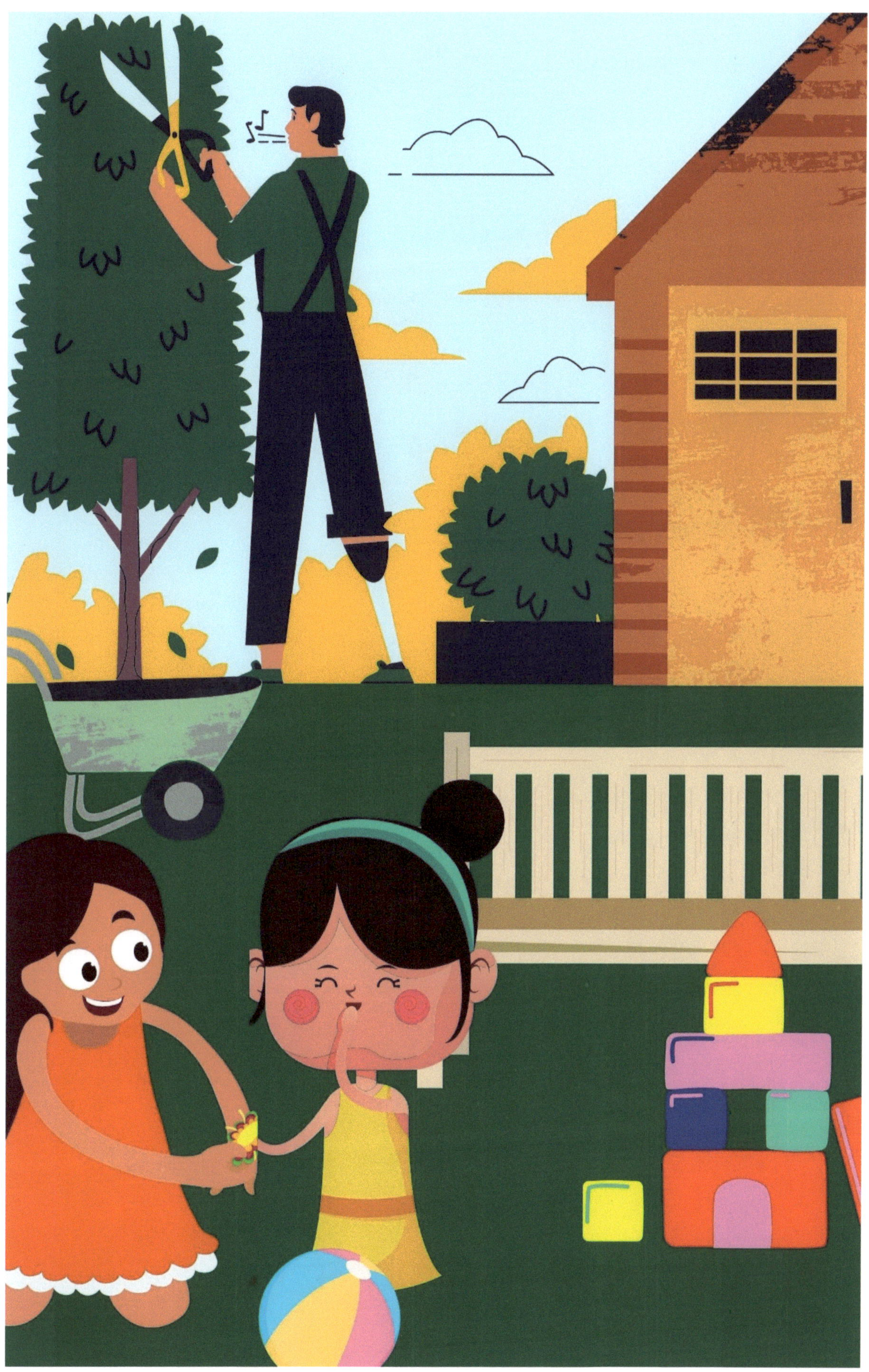

Jana at the hospital

Jana at the hospital

Oftentimes, we'll find that parents don't know what to say to their child about surgery, for instance, so they don't tell them anything.

This story has several qualities: accurate information, a suitable balance of words and images, and an age-appropriate yet honest approach to the subject matter.

This book is available in several languages: English, French, Arabic.

Jana at the hospital

Jana at the hospital

Jana at the hospital